44 Asthma Reducing Juice Recipes:

Home Remedies for Asthmatic Patients Who Want Fast and Instant Relief

By

Joe Correa CSN

COPYRIGHT

This publication is designed to provide accurate and authoritative information in regard to the subject matter covered. It is sold with the understanding that neither the author nor the publisher is engaged in rendering medical advice. If medical advice or assistance is needed, consult with a doctor. This book is considered a guide and should not be used in any way detrimental to your health. Consult with a physician before starting this nutritional plan to make sure it's right for you.

ACKNOWLEDGEMENTS

This book is dedicated to my friends and family that have had mild or serious illnesses so that you may find a solution and make the necessary changes in your life.

44 Asthma Reducing Juice Recipes:

Home Remedies for Asthmatic Patients Who Want Fast and Instant Relief

By

Joe Correa CSN

CONTENTS

ABOUT THE AUTHOR

After years of Research, I honestly believe in the positive effects that proper nutrition can have over the body and mind. My knowledge and experience has helped me live healthier throughout the years and which I have shared with family and friends. The more you know about eating and drinking healthier, the sooner you will want to change your life and eating habits.

Nutrition is a key part in the process of being healthy and living longer so get started today. The first step is the most important and the most significant.

INTRODUCTION

44 Asthma Reducing Juice Recipes: Home Remedies for Asthmatic Patients Who Want Fast and Instant Relief

By Joe Correa CSN

Asthma is a chronic lung disease in which your airways narrow and swell making breathing difficult and causing shortness of breath and coughing. In some cases, asthma is a minor discomfort while in others it can be a major problem and a life-threatening condition.

Symptoms of asthma vary from person to person and depend on the condition itself. Some common signs include regular shortness of breath, unexplainable chest pain, sleep problems caused by coughing, wheezing or shortness of breath, whistling sound when exhaling.

The cure for asthma still doesn't exist but the symptoms can be controlled with regular treatment. If you notice any of the described symptoms, it's extremely important to make an appointment with your physician. An early treatment of asthma may prevent long-term lung damage this disease may cause. Your doctor will help you keep it under control by monitoring the condition after its diagnosis.

In some cases, people who have been diagnosed with asthma may experience a rapid worsening of symptoms with no improvement even after using medication. In such cases, an emergency treatment can save your life.

There are several factors that can trigger symptoms of asthma and vary from person to person. These triggers include:

- Respiratory infections
- Cold air and air pollutants like smoke
- Different medications
- Preservatives added to food and beverages
- Stress and strong emotions
- Polled, dust mites, mold spores, and other air substances
- Excessive use of cigarettes or exposure to secondhand smoke

Avoiding these common triggers will significantly reduce the risk of asthma. Furthermore, there are certain types of foods that are proven to help prevent and treat people diagnosed with asthma. Vitamin D rich foods like milk and eggs are often prescribed to patients suffering from asthma. Also, vegetables rich in beta-carotene such as carrots, bell peppers, pumpkin, and leafy greens are proven to be extremely beneficial for reducing the risk of asthma. Furthermore, some studies suggest that people with low magnesium levels have low lung volume. Adding foods rich in magnesium into your diet is an excellent way to prevent and treat asthma attacks.

This book contains asthma preventing juice recipes based on these particular foods that will help you reduce the risk of getting asthma in the first place. The juices in this book are very easy to make, healthy, and above all, delicious.

44 ASTHMA REDUCING JUICE RECIPES: HOME REMEDIES FOR ASTHMATIC PATIENTS WHO WANT FAST AND INSTANT RELIEF

1. Broccoli Cauliflower Juice

Ingredients:

1 cup broccoli, chopped

1 cup cauliflower, chopped

1 small Granny Smith's apple, cored

1 cup fresh kale, torn

¼ tsp ginger, ground

Preparation:

Wash the broccoli thoroughly and chop into small pieces. Set aside.

Wash the cauliflower and trim off the outer leaves. Cut into small pieces and set aside.

Wash the apple and cut lengthwise in half. Remove the core and cut into bite-sized pieces. Set aside.

Rinse the kale under cold running water and slightly drain. Torn with hands and set aside.

Now, combine broccoli, cauliflower, apple, and kale in a juicer and process until well juiced. Transfer to a serving glass and stir in the ground ginger.

Refrigerate for 10-15 minutes before serving.

Nutritional information per serving: Kcal: 131, Protein: 8.1g, Carbs: 36.8g, Fats: 1.5g

2. Apple Carrot Juice

Ingredients:

1 large Zestar apple, cored

1 medium-sized carrot, chopped

1 whole lemon, peeled

1 large peach, pitted

¼ tsp cinnamon, ground

2 oz water

Preparation:

Wash the apple and cut lengthwise in half. Remove the core and cut into bite-sized pieces. Set aside.

Wash and peel the carrot. Cut into small chunks and set aside.

Peel the lemon and cut lengthwise in half. Set aside.

Wash the peach and cut in half. Remove the pit and cut into bite-sized pieces. Set aside.

Now, combine apple, carrot lemon, and peach in a juicer. Process until nicely juiced. Transfer to a serving glass and stir in the water and cinnamon.

Add a few ice cubes and serve immediately.

Enjoy!

Nutritional information per serving: Kcal: 165, Protein: 3.6g, Carbs: 50.7g, Fats: 1.1g

3. Orange Raspberry Juice

Ingredients:

1 large orange, wedged

1 cup raspberries

2 large carrots, peeled and chopped

¼ tsp ginger, ground

1 tbsp liquid honey

Preparation:

Peel the orange and divide into wedges. Set aside.

Using a colander, rinse the raspberries under cold running water and drain. Set aside.

Wash the carrots and peel them. Cut into small chunks and set aside.

Now, combine orange, raspberries, and carrots in a juicer and process until well juiced. Transfer to a serving glass and stir in the ginger and honey.

Let it chill in the refrigerator for a while before serving.

Nutritional information per serving: Kcal: 204, Protein: 4.5g, Carbs: 67.1g, Fats: 1.3g

4. Beet Broccoli Juice

Ingredients:

1 whole beet, chopped

1 cup broccoli, chopped

1 cup purple cabbage, torn

1 cup Swiss chard, torn

1 cup cucumber, sliced

¼ tsp turmeric, ground

Preparation:

Wash the beets and trim off the green parts. Cut into bite-sized pieces and set aside.

Wash the broccoli and trim off the outer layers. Chop it into small pieces and set aside.

Combine purple cabbage and Swiss chard in a large colander. Wash thoroughly under cold running water and slightly drain. Torn with hands and set aside.

Wash the cucumber and cut into thin slices. Fill the measuring cup and reserve the rest for later. Set aside.

Now, combine beet, broccoli, purple cabbage, Swiss chard,

and cucumber in a juicer and process until juiced.

Transfer to a serving glass and stir in the turmeric. Refrigerate for 10 minutes and serve.

Enjoy!

Nutrition information per serving: Kcal: 79, Protein: 6.2g, Carbs: 23.7g, Fats: 0.8g

5. Cucumber Agave Juice

Ingredients:

1 cup cucumber, sliced

1 tsp agave nectar

1 cup cauliflower, chopped

1 cup fresh kale, chopped

1 whole lime, peeled

Preparation:

Wash the cucumber and cut into thin slices. Fill the measuring cup and reserve the rest for some other juice. Set aside.

Wash the kale thoroughly under cold running water and slightly drain. Chop into small pieces and set aside.

Peel the lime and cut lengthwise in half. Set aside.

Trim off the outer layer of the cauliflower. Cut into bite-sized pieces and wash it. Fill the measuring cup and sprinkle with some salt. Set aside.

Now, combine cucumber, kale, lime, and cauliflower in a juicer. Process until well juiced. Transfer to a serving glass and stir in the agave nectar.

Refrigerate before serving.

Enjoy!

Nutrition information per serving: Kcal: 107, Protein: 11.4g, Carbs: 30.4g, Fats: 1.8g

6. Lemon Apple Juice

Ingredients:

1 whole lemon, peeled

1 medium-sized Zestar apple, cored

1 cup raspberries

1 cup fresh mint, torn

1 cup cranberries

¼ tsp cinnamon, ground

Preparation:

Peel the lemon and cut lengthwise in half. Set aside.

Wash the apple and cut in half. Remove the core and cut into bite-sized pieces.

Combine raspberries and cranberries in a large colander. Rinse thoroughly under cold running water and slightly drain. Set aside.

Rinse the mint and torn with hands. Set aside.

Now, combine lemon, apple, raspberries, mint, and cranberries in a juicer and process until juiced. Transfer to a serving glass and stir in the cinnamon. Add some ice before serving.

Enjoy!

Nutrition information per serving: Kcal: 143, Protein: 3.8g, Carbs: 53.5g, Fats: 1.5g

7. Avocado Lemon Juice

Ingredients:

1 cup avocado, cubed

1 whole lemon, peeled

2 whole plums, chopped

1 medium-sized Granny Smith's apple, cored

¼ tsp cinnamon, ground

1 tbsp coconut water

Preparation:

Peel the avocado and cut in half. Remove the pit and cut into small cubes. Fill the measuring cup and reserve the rest for later.

Peel the lemon and cut into half. Set aside.

Wash the plums and cut lengthwise in half. Remove the pits and cut into bite-sized pieces. Set aside.

Wash the apple and cut in half. Remove the pit and cut into small pieces. Set aside.

Now, combine avocado, lemon plums, and apple in a juicer and process until juiced. Transfer to a serving glass and stir in the cinnamon and coconut water.

Refrigerate for 15 minutes before serving.

Enjoy!

Nutrition information per serving: Kcal: 341, Protein: 5.3g, Carbs: 56.1g, Fats: 22.8g

8. Lemon Strawberry Juice

Ingredients:

1 medium-sized pear, chopped

1 cup blueberries

1 whole lemon, peeled

½ cup strawberries, sliced

1 small ginger knob, peeled

1 oz water

Preparation:

Peel the lemon and cut in half. Set aside.

Wash the strawberries and remove the stems. Cut into small pieces and fill the measuring cup. Set aside.

Wash the pear and cut in half. Remove the core and cut into small pieces. Set aside.

Rinse the blueberries and fill the measuring cup. Set aside.

Peel the ginger knob and set aside.

Now, combine lemon, strawberries, pear, blueberries, and ginger in a juicer and process until juiced. Transfer to a serving glass and stir in the water.

Serve immediately.

Nutritional information per serving: Kcal: 143, Protein: 2.4g, Carbs: 52.7g, Fats: 0.8g

9. Cinnamon Watermelon Juice

Ingredients:

¼ tsp cinnamon, ground

1 medium-sized watermelon wedge

1 large banana, peeled

1 whole lime, peeled

1 small Granny Smith's apple, cored

Preparation:

Cut one large watermelon wedge and peel it. Remove the seeds and cut into bite-sized pieces. Wrap the rest of the melon in a plastic foil and refrigerate.

Peel the banana and chop into small chunks. Set aside.

Peel the lime and cut lengthwise in half. Set aside.

Wash the apple and cut in half. Remove the core and cut into bite-sized pieces. Set aside.

Now, combine watermelon, lime, banana, and apple in a juicer and process until juiced. Transfer to a serving glass and stir in the cinnamon.

Refrigerate for 10 minutes before serving.

Nutritional information per serving: Kcal: 226, Protein: 4.6g, Carbs: 29.4g, Fats: 1.2g

10. Lemon Artichoke Juice

Ingredients:

1 whole lemon, peeled

1 medium-sized artichoke, chopped

1 large blood orange, peeled

1 whole lime, peeled

1 tbsp liquid honey

1 oz water

Preparation:

Peel the lemon and lime. Cut each fruit lengthwise in half and set aside.

Trim off the outer layers of the artichoke using a sharp paring knife. Cut into bite-sized pieces and set aside.

Peel the orange and divide into wedges. Cut each wedge in half and set aside.

Now, combine lemon, artichoke, orange, and lime in a juicer. Process until well juiced. Transfer to a serving glass and stir in the honey and water.

Refrigerate for 10 minutes before serving.

Nutrition information per serving: Kcal: 149, Protein: 5.9g, Carbs: 33.8g, Fats: 0.5g

11. Apple Vanilla Juice

Ingredients:

1 small Red Delicious apple, cored

¼ tsp vanilla extract

1 cup blueberries

1 whole grapefruit, peeled

1 cup avocado, cubed

Preparation:

Wash the apple and cut lengthwise in half. Remove the core and cut into bite-sized pieces. Set aside.

Place the blueberries in a colander. Rinse well under cold running water and drain. Set aside.

Peel the grapefruit and divide into wedges. Cut each wedge in half and set aside.

Peel the avocado and cut lengthwise in half. Remove the pit and cut into small cubes. Fill the measuring cup and reserve the rest in the refrigerator.

Now, combine apple, blueberries, grapefruit, and avocado in a juicer and process until juiced. Transfer to a serving glass and stir in the vanilla extract. Refrigerate for 10 minutes before serving.

Nutrition information per serving: Kcal: 436, Protein: 6.4g, Carbs: 69.5g, Fats: 23.2g

12. Banana Pineapple Juice

Ingredients:

1 large banana, chunked

1 cup pineapple, chunked

1 cup strawberries, chopped

1 whole lemon, peeled

1 tbsp fresh mint, finely chopped

Preparation:

Peel the banana and cut into small chunks. Set aside.

Cut the top of the pineapple using a sharp paring knife. Gently remove all hard skin and slice it into thin slices. Fill the measuring cup and reserve the rest for later.

Wash the strawberries and remove the stems. Chop into small pieces and fill the measuring cup. Reserve the rest in the refrigerator.

Peel the lemon and cut lengthwise in half. Set aside.

Now, combine banana, pineapple, strawberries, and lemon in a juicer. Process until juiced. Transfer to a serving glass and stir in the mint.

Add few ice cubes and serve immediately.

Nutrition information per serving: Kcal: 224, Protein: 4.1g, Carbs: 69.4g, Fats: 1.3g

13. Blueberry Coconut Juice

Ingredients:

2 cups blueberries

2 oz coconut water

1 large honeydew melon wedge, chopped

1 medium-sized Zestar apple, cored

1 tbsp mint, finely chopped

Preparation:

Place the blueberries in a large colander. Rinse well under cold running water and drain. Set aside.

Cut melon lengthwise in half. Scoop out the seeds and then wash. Cut one large wedge and peel it. Cut into small cubes and set aside.

Wash the apple and cut lengthwise in half. Remove the core and cut into bite-sized pieces. Set aside.

Now, combine blueberry, honeydew melon, apple in a juicer. Process until juiced.

Transfer to a serving glass and stir in the coconut water and mint. Add some crushed ice and serve immediately.

Nutrition information per serving: Kcal: 283, Protein: 3.7g, Carbs: 85.1g, Fats: 1.5g

14. Lime Cauliflower Juice

Ingredients:

1 large lime, peeled

1 cup cauliflower, chopped

3 large leeks, chopped

1 large zucchini, chopped

2 oz water

Preparation:

Peel the lime and cut lengthwise in half. Set aside.

Trim off the outer leaves of cauliflower. Wash it and cut into small pieces. Set aside.

Wash the leeks and cut into small pieces. Set aside.

Peel the zucchini and cut in half. Scrape out the seeds and cut into small chunks. Set aside.

Now, combine lime, cauliflower, leeks, and zucchini in a juicer. Process until well juiced and stir in the water. Refrigerate for 10 minutes before serving.

Enjoy!

Nutritional information per serving: Kcal: 241, Protein: 13.2g, Carbs: 64.7g, Fats: 2.6g

15. Apple Strawberry Juice

Ingredients:

1 large Red Delicious apple, cored

1 cup strawberries, chopped

2 large peaches, pitted

1 large lemon, peeled

1 large kiwi, peeled

1 large orange, peeled

2 oz water

Preparation:

Wash the apple and cut half. Remove the core and cut into bite-sized pieces. Set aside.

Wash the strawberries under cold running water. Remove the green parts and cut into bite-sized pieces. Set aside.

Wash the peaches and cut in half. Remove the pits and cut into small pieces. Set aside.

Peel the lemon and kiwi. Cut lengthwise in half and set aside.

Peel the orange and divide into wedges. Set aside.

Now, combine apple, strawberries, peaches, lemon, kiwi, and orange in a juicer and process until well juiced. Transfer to serving glasses and stir in the water. Add some ice and serve immediately.

Enjoy!

Nutritional information per serving: Kcal: 345, Protein: 7.8g, Carbs: 105g, Fats: 2.3g

16. Carrot Watercress Juice

Ingredients:

2 large carrots, sliced

1 cup watercress, torn

1 cup pineapple, chunked

1 large lime, peeled

1 small ginger knob, peeled

2 oz water

Preparation:

Wash and peel the carrots. Cut into thin slices and set aside.

Wash the watercress thoroughly under cold running water. Torn with hands and set aside.

Peel the pineapple and cut into small chunks. Set aside.

Peel the lime and cut lengthwise in half. Set aside.

Peel the ginger root knob and cut into small pieces. Set aside.

Now, combine carrots, watercress, pineapple, lemon, and

ginger in a juicer and process until well juiced.

Transfer to serving glasses and stir in water.

Add some ice and serve.

Nutritional information per serving: Kcal: 135, Protein: 3.3g, Carbs: 40.6g, Fats: 3.3g

17. Pomegranate Orange Juice

Ingredients:

1 cup pomegranate seeds

2 large oranges, peeled

2 large apricots, pitted

1 cup green grapes

1 large lemon, peeled

1 small ginger slice, peeled

Preparation:

Cut the top of the pomegranate fruit using a sharp knife. Slice down to each of the white membranes inside of the fruit. Pop the seeds into a measuring cup and set aside.

Peel the oranges and divide into wedges. Set aside.

Wash the apricots and cut in half. Remove the pits and cut into small pieces. Set aside.

Rinse the grapes and fill the measuring cup. Reserve the rest in the refrigerator.

Peel the lemon and cut lengthwise in half. Set aside.

Peel the ginger slice and set aside.

Now, combine pomegranate, oranges, grapes, apricots, lemon, and ginger in a juicer. Process until well juiced and transfer to serving glasses. Refrigerate for 10 minutes before serving.

Nutritional information per serving: Kcal: 294, Protein: 7.2g, Carbs: 88.9g, Fats: 2.3g

18. Mint Papaya Juice

Ingredients:

1 tbsp fresh mint, chopped

1 large papaya, peeled and chopped

1 large Red Delicious apple, cored

1 cup pomegranate seeds

2 oz water

Preparation:

Peel the papaya and cut lengthwise in half. Scoop out the black seeds and flesh using a spoon. Cut into small chunks and set aside.

Wash the apple and cut in half. Using a sharp knife, remove the core and cut into bite-sized pieces. Set aside.

Cut the top of the pomegranate fruit using a sharp knife. Slice down to each of the white membranes inside of the fruit. Pop the seeds into a measuring cup and set aside.

Now, combine mint, papaya, apple, and pomegranate in a juicer. Process until well juiced and transfer to serving glasses. Stir in the water and refrigerate before serving.

Nutritional information per serving: Kcal: 438, Protein: 6.1g, Carbs: 129g, Fats: 3.4g

19. Beet Mint Juice

Ingredients:

1 cup beets, chopped

1 cup fresh mint, torn

2 cups raspberries

1 large Red Delicious apple, cored

1 large lemon, peeled

3 oz water

Preparation:

Wash the beets and trim off the green ends. Cut into small pieces and fill the measuring cup. Reserve the greens for some other juice.

Wash the raspberries under cold running water using a colander. Drain and set aside.

Wash the apple and cut in half. Remove the core and cut into bite-sized pieces. Set aside.

Rinse the mint thoroughly under cold running water and torn with hands. Set aside.

Peel the lemon and cut lengthwise in half. Set aside.

Now, combine beets, mint, raspberries, apple, and lemon in a juicer. Process until well juiced. Stir in the water and refrigerate for 15 minutes before serving.

Enjoy!

Nutritional information per serving: Kcal: 218, Protein: 7.5g, Carbs: 76.4g, Fats: 2.5g

20. Pumpkin Swiss Chard Juice

Ingredients:

2 cups pumpkin, cubed

1 cup Swiss chard, torn

1 large Granny Smith's apple, cored

¼ tsp cinnamon, ground

1 large cucumber, sliced

2 oz water

Preparation:

Peel the pumpkin and cut in half. Scoop out the seeds using a spoon. Cut one large wedge and peel it. Cut into small cubes and fill the measuring cup. Reserve the rest for some other juice.

Wash the Swiss chard thoroughly under cold running water. Drain and torn with hands. Set aside.

Wash the apple and cut in half. Remove the core and cut into bite-sized pieces. Set aside.

Wash the cucumber and cut into thin slices. Set aside.

Now, combine pumpkin, Swiss chard, apple, and cucumber

in a juicer. Process until well juiced and stir in the water and nutmeg.

Refrigerate for 10 minutes before serving.

Nutritional information per serving: Kcal: 196, Protein: 5.8g, Carbs: 55.4g, Fats: 1.1g

21. Watermelon Mint Juice

Ingredients:

1 cup watermelon, cubed

1 cup fresh mint, torn

2 cups blueberries

1 whole lime, peeled

¼ tsp cayenne pepper, ground

1 oz water

Preparation:

Cut one large watermelon wedge. Using a sharp paring knife, peel and cut into small cubes. Remove the seeds and set aside.

Rinse the mint and roughly torn it with hands. Set aside.

Place the blueberries in a large colander. Rinse well under cold running water and set aside.

Peel the lime and cut lengthwise in half. Set aside.

Now, combine watermelon, mint, blueberries, and lime in a juicer. Process until juiced. Transfer to a serving glass and stir in the cayenne pepper and water.

Refrigerate for 5 minutes before serving.

Nutritional information per serving: Kcal: 198, Protein: 4.1g, Carbs: 58.7g, Fats: 1.4g

22. Cherry Lemon Juice

Ingredients:

1 cup cherries, pitted

1 whole lemon, peeled

1 cup pineapple, chunked

1 cup spinach, chopped

¼ tsp cinnamon, ground

1 oz water

Preparation:

Place the cherries in a medium colander. Rinse well under cold running water and remove the stems, if any. Cut each in half and remove the pits. Fill the measuring cup and reserve the rest in the refrigerator.

Peel the lemon and cut lengthwise in half. Set aside.

Using a sharp paring knife, cut the top of the pineapple. Gently remove all hard skin and slice it into thin slices. Fill the measuring cup and reserve the rest for later.

Rinse the spinach thoroughly under cold running water. Drain and chop into small pieces. Set aside.

Now, combine cherries, lemon pineapple, and spinach in a juicer and process until juiced. Transfer to a serving glass and stir in the water.

Add some crushed ice and serve immediately.

Nutrition information per serving: Kcal: 196, Protein: 9.2g, Carbs: 59.3g, Fats: 1.5g

23. Apricot Honey Juice

Ingredients:

1 cup of apricots, pitted and halved

1 tbsp liquid honey

1 small pear, chopped

1 whole lemon, peeled and halved

1 small Granny Smith's apple, cored

1 cup fresh mint, torn

Preparation:

Wash the apricots and cut each lengthwise in half. Remove the pits and fill the measuring cup. Reserve the rest in the refrigerator for some other juice.

Wash the pear and cut in half. Remove the core and cut into small pieces. Set aside.

Peel the lemon and cut lengthwise in half. Set aside.

Wash the apple and cut lengthwise in half. Remove the core and chop into bite-sized pieces. Set aside.

Rinse the mint thoroughly under cold running water. Drain and torn into small pieces. Set aside.

Now, combine apricots, apple, pear, lemon, and mint in a juicer and process until well juiced. Transfer to a serving glass and add some ice before serving.

Enjoy!

Nutrition information per serving: Kcal: 217, Protein: 4.9g, Carbs: 68.5g, Fats: 1.5g

24. Celery Ginger Juice

Ingredients:

1 cup celery, chopped

1 whole kiwi, peeled

1 medium-sized Golden Delicious apple, cored

1 medium-sized orange, peeled

1 tbsp liquid honey

¼ tsp ginger, ground

Preparation:

Wash the celery and chop into small pieces. Fill the measuring cup and reserve the rest for later. Set aside.

Peel the kiwi and cut lengthwise in half. Set aside.

Wash the apple and cut lengthwise in half. Remove the core and cut into bite-sized pieces. Set aside.

Peel the orange and divide into wedges. Cut each wedge in half and set aside.

Now, combine kiwi, apple, celery, and orange in a juicer and process until juiced. Transfer to a serving glass and stir in the honey and ginger.

Refrigerate for 15 minutes before serving.

Enjoy!

Nutrition information per serving: Kcal: 172, Protein: 3.5g, Carbs: 51.2g, Fats: 1.1g

25. Apricot Orange Juice

Ingredients:

1 large apricot, pitted

1 large orange, wedged

1 cup pomegranate seeds

1 large lemon, peeled

1 large carrot, sliced

2 oz coconut water

Preparation:

Wash the apricot and cut in half. Remove the pit and cut into small pieces. Set aside.

Peel the orange and divide into wedges. Set aside.

Cut the top of the pomegranate fruit using a sharp knife. Slice down to each of the white membranes inside of the fruit. Pop the seeds into measuring cup and set aside.

Peel the lemon and cut lengthwise in half. Set aside.

Peel and wash the carrot. Cut into thin slices and set aside.

Now, combine apricot, orange, pomegranate seeds, lemon,

and carrot in a juicer. Process until well juiced and transfer to serving glasses. Stir in the coconut water and add few ice cubes before serving.

Nutritional information per serving: Kcal: 241, Protein: 7.3g, Carbs: 73.9g, Fats: 2.3g

26. Orange Pineapple Juice

Ingredients:

1 large orange, peeled

1 cup pineapple, chunked

1 whole grapefruit, peeled

1 cup cauliflower, chopped

¼ cup pure coconut water, unsweetened

Preparation:

Peel the orange and grapefruit and divide into wedges. Set aside.

Cut the top of a pineapple and peel it using a sharp knife. Cut into small chunks. Reserve the rest of the pineapple in a refrigerator.

Trim off the outer leaves of cauliflower. Wash it and cut into small pieces. Reserve the rest in the refrigerator.

Now, combine orange, pineapple, grapefruit, and cauliflower in a juicer and process until juiced. Transfer to serving glasses and stir in the pure coconut water.

Add few ice cubes and serve immediately.

Nutritional information per serving: Kcal: 247, Protein: 6.5g, Carbs: 74g, Fats: 1g

27. Cantaloupe Orange Juice

Ingredients:

1 cup cantaloupe, chopped

1 large orange, peeled

1 cup blackberries

1 cup fresh mint, torn

¼ tsp cinnamon, ground

Preparation:

Cut the cantaloupe in half. Scrape out the seeds and cut one large wedge. Peel and chop into small pieces. Fill the measuring cup and wrap the rest in a plastic foil. Refrigerate for later.

Peel the orange and divide into wedges. Cut each wedge in half and set aside.

Place the blackberries in a colander and rinse well. Drain and set aside.

Rinse the mint under cold running water and drain. Torn into small pieces and set aside.

Now, combine cantaloupe, orange blackberries, and mint

in a juicer and process until juiced. Transfer to a serving glass and stir in the cinnamon. Optionally, add some water to increase the juice amount.

Serve immediately.

Nutrition information per serving: Kcal: 157, Protein: 5.9g, Carbs: 51.9g, Fats: 1.5g

28. Cucumber Apple Juice

Ingredients:

1 medium-sized cucumber, chopped

1 small Golden Delicious apple, cored

1 large honeydew melon wedge, chopped

1 cup fresh mint, chopped

1 oz coconut water

Preparation:

Wash the cucumber and cut into thin slices. Set aside.

Wash the apple and cut lengthwise in half. Remove the core and cut into bite-sized pieces. Set aside.

Cut the melon in half. Cut one large wedge and peel the peel it. Cut into small pieces and set aside. Wrap the rest of the melon in a plastic foil and refrigerate for later.

Place mint in a colander and wash thoroughly. Slightly drain and chop into small pieces. Set aside.

Now, combine cucumber, apple, melon, and mint in a juicer and process until juiced.

Transfer to a serving glass and stir in the water. Optionally, add 1 tablespoon of lemon juice for a better taste. Refrigerate for 10 minutes before serving.

Enjoy!

Nutrition information per serving: Kcal: 139, Protein: 4.1g, Carbs: 40.5g, Fats: 0.9g

29. Watermelon Celery Juice

Ingredients:

1 medium-sized watermelon slice

1 cup celery, chopped

2 cups cherries, pitted

1 small ginger knob, peeled

1 oz water

Preparation:

Cut the watermelon in half. Cut one medium-sized wedge and wrap the rest in a plastic foil and refrigerate. Dice the wedge and remove the pits. Set aside.

Wash the celery and cut into small pieces. Fill the measuring cup and reserve the rest for later. Set aside.

Rinse the cherries under cold running water using a colander. Drain and cut each in half. Remove the pits and set aside.

Peel the ginger knob and cut into small pieces. Set aside.

Now, combine watermelon, celery, cherries, and ginger knob in a juicer and process until juiced. Transfer to a serving glass and stir in the water. Optionally, you can use coconut water if you like.

Serve immediately.

Nutrition information per serving: Kcal: 143, Protein: 3.4g, Carbs: 40.2g, Fats: 0.7g

30. Apple Carrot Juice

Ingredients:

3 medium-sized carrots, sliced

1 cup parsnips, sliced

2 large Gala apples, peeled and cored

¼ cup water

1 tbsp fresh lemon juice

Preparation:

Wash the carrots and parsnips and cut into thick slices. Set aside.

Wash the apples and remove the core. Cut into bite-sized pieces and set aside.

Now, combine apples, carrots, and parsnips in a juicer and process until juiced.

Transfer to serving glasses and stir in the water and lemon juice. Garnish with some mint and refrigerate before serving.

Enjoy!

Nutritional information per serving: Kcal: 332, Protein: 5.4g, Carbs: 100g, Fats: 1.6g

31. Cabbage Grapefruit Juice

Ingredients:

2 whole kiwis, peeled

1 cup carrots, chopped

2 cups green cabbage, shredded

1 whole grapefruit, peeled

1 tbsp honey, raw

Preparation:

Wash the cabbage thoroughly and roughly chop it using hands. Set aside.

Wash the grapefruit and cut into chunks. Set aside.

Wash the carrots and cut into small pieces. Set aside.

Peel the kiwis and cut in half. Set aside.

Now, process cabbage, grapefruit, carrots, and kiwis in a juicer. Transfer to a serving glass and stir in the honey.

Serve immediately.

Nutritional information per serving: Kcal: 219, Protein: 6.9g, Carbs: 69g, Fats: 1.5g

32. Cantaloupe Kale Juice

Ingredients:

1 cup cantaloupe, cubed

1 cup fresh kale, torn

1 small Red Delicious apple, cored

1 cup beets, sliced

¼ tsp ginger, ground

Preparation:

Cut the cantaloupe in half. Scrape out the seeds and cut one large wedge. Peel and chop into small pieces. Fill the measuring cup and wrap the rest in a plastic foil. Refrigerate for later.

Rinse the kale thoroughly under cold running water. Drain and torn into small pieces. Set aside.

Wash the apple and cut lengthwise in half. Remove the core and cut into bite-sized pieces. Set aside.

Wash the beets and trim off the green ends. Cut into thin slices and fill the measuring cup. Reserve the rest for some other juice.

Now, combine cantaloupe, kale, apple, and beets in a juicer and process until juiced. Transfer to a serving glass and stir in the ginger.

Add some ice and serve immediately.

Nutrition information per serving: Kcal: 181, Protein: 7g, Carbs: 51.1g, Fats: 1.4g

33. Carrot Apple Juice

Ingredients:

1 cup mango, chunked

1 medium-sized orange, wedged

1 large carrot, sliced

1 small Granny Smith's apple, cored and chopped

1 oz coconut water

Preparation:

Peel the mango and cut into chunks. Fill the measuring cup and reserve the rest for later.

Peel the orange and divide into wedges. Set aside.

Wash and peel the carrot. Cut into bite-sized pieces and set aside.

Wash the apple and cut in half. Remove the core and cut into bite-sized pieces. Set aside.

Now, combine mango, orange, carrot, and apple in a juicer and process until juiced. Transfer to a serving glass and stir in the coconut water.

Serve immediately and enjoy!

Nutrition information per serving: Kcal: 189, Protein: 2.6g, Carbs: 56.4g, Fats:1.1g

34. Lime Melon Juice

Ingredients:

1 large lime, peeled

2 large honeydew melon wedges

1 cup avocado, peeled and pitted

5 tbsp fresh mint

1 medium-sized pineapple slice, chopped

Preparation:

Peel the lime and cut lengthwise in half. Set aside.

Cut the honeydew melon lengthwise in half. Scoop out the seeds using a spoon. Cut the large wedges and peel them. Cut into small chunks and place in a bowl. Wrap the rest of the melon in a plastic foil and refrigerate.

Peel the avocado and cut in half. Remove the pit and cut into chunks. Add it to the bowl with melon and set aside.

Wash the mint leaves and soak in water for 5 minutes.

Now, process lime, honeydew melon, avocado, mint, and pineapple in a juicer. Transfer to serving glasses and serve immediately.

Enjoy!

Nutritional information per serving: Kcal: 321, Protein: 5.2g, Carbs: 46.8g, Fats: 22.6g

35. Pomegranate Kale Juice

Ingredients:

½ cup pomegranate seeds

½ cup fresh kale, torn

1 tsp fresh ginger, freshly grated

1 large Granny Smith's apple, cored

1 tbsp agave nectar

Preparation:

Cut the top of the pomegranate fruit using a sharp knife. slice down to each of the white membranes inside of the fruit. Pop the seeds into a medium-sized bowl.

Rinse the kale thoroughly. Drain and torn into small pieces. Set aside.

Peel and grate the ginger knob. Fill up the measuring teaspoon and reserve the rest in the refrigerator.

Wash the apple and remove the core. Cut into bite-sized pieces and set aside.

Process the pomegranate seeds, kale, and apple in a juicer until well juiced.

Transfer to serving glasses and stir in the ginger. Add some water to adjust the thickness and stir in the agave nectar.

Serve immediately.

Nutrition information per serving: Kcal: 194, Protein: 6.2g, Carbs: 54.2g, Fats: 2.4g

36. Spinach Avocado Juice

Ingredients:

1 cup fresh spinach, torn

1 cup avocado, cubed

1 cup artichoke, chopped

1 cup green cabbage, torn

¼ tsp ginger powder

Preparation:

Combine spinach and cabbage in a large colander. Wash thoroughly under cold running water. Drain and torn into small pieces. Set aside.

Peel the avocado and cut lengthwise in half. Remove the pit and cut into small cubes. Fill the measuring cup and reserve the rest in the refrigerator.

Trim off the outer layers of the artichoke using a sharp paring knife. Cut into bite-sized pieces and fill the measuring cup. Reserve the rest for later.

Now, combine spinach, avocado, artichoke, and cabbage in a juicer and process until juiced. Transfer to a serving glass and stir in the ginger powder.

Refrigerate for 15 minutes before serving.

Nutrition information per serving: Kcal: 282, Protein: 15.4g, Carbs: 42.6g, Fats: 23.2g

37. Cantaloupe Mint Juice

Ingredients:

1 cup cantaloupe, chopped

1 cup fresh mint, torn

1 whole plum, chopped

1 large orange, peeled

¼ tsp ginger, ground

Preparation:

Cut the cantaloupe in half. Scoop out the seeds and flesh. Cut and peel one large wedge. Chop into chunks and fill the measuring cup. Reserve the rest of the cantaloupe in a refrigerator.

Wash the mint thoroughly under cold running water. Torn into small pieces and set aside.

Peel the orange and divide into wedges. Cut each wedge in half and set aside.

Wash the plum and cut in half. Remove the pit and chop into small pieces. Set aside.

Now, combine cantaloupe, mint, plum, and orange in a

juicer and process until juiced. Transfer to a serving glass and stir in the ginger.

Serve immediately.

Nutrition information per serving: Kcal: 151, Protein: 4.4g, Carbs: 45.6g, Fats: 0.9g

38. Pomegranate Plum Juice

Ingredients:

1 cup pomegranate seeds

3 whole plums, pitted and chopped

1 cup yellow pumpkin, cubed

1 medium-sized orange, peeled

¼ tsp ginger, ground

1 oz water

Preparation:

Cut the top of the pomegranate fruit using a sharp paring knife. Slice down to each of the white membranes inside of the fruit. Pop the seeds into a measuring cup and set aside.

Wash the plums and cut into halves. Remove the pits and chop into small pieces. Set aside.

Cut the top of a pumpkin. Cut lengthwise in half and then scrape out the seeds. Cut one large wedge and peel it. Cut into small cubes and fill the measuring cup. Reserve the rest in the refrigerator.

Peel the orange and divide into wedges. Cut each wedge in

half and set aside.

Now, combine pomegranate, plums, pumpkin, and orange in a juicer. Process until juiced. Transfer to a serving glass and stir in the ginger and water.

Refrigerate for 15 minutes before serving.

Enjoy!
Nutrition information per serving: Kcal: 214, Protein: 5.2g, Carbs: 61.8g, Fats: 1.8g

39. Strawberry Grapefruit Juice

Ingredients:

2 large strawberries, chopped

2 large grapefruits, peeled

1 large Red Delicious apple, cored

1 small ginger knob, peeled

2 oz coconut water

Preparation:

Wash the strawberries and cut into small pieces. Set aside.

Peel the grapefruits and divide into wedges. Set aside.

Wash the apple and cut in half. Remove the core and cut into bite-sized pieces. Set aside.

Peel the ginger knob and set aside.

Now, combine strawberries, grapefruits, apple, and ginger in a juicer. Process until well juiced and transfer to serving glasses. Stir in the coconut water and refrigerate for 15 minutes, or add some ice before serving.

Nutritional information per serving: Kcal: 302, Protein: 4.8g, Carbs: 86.3g, Fats: 1.7g

40. Lime Zucchini Juice

Ingredients:

1 large lime, peeled

1 large zucchini, seeded

3 large kiwis, peeled

1 cup pomegranate seeds

1 large orange, peeled

Preparation:

Peel the lime and kiwi. Cut lengthwise in half and set aside.

Wash the zucchini and cut in half. Scoop out the seeds using a spoon. Cut into small chunks and set aside.

Cut the top of the pomegranate fruit using a sharp knife. Slice down to each of the white membranes inside of the fruit. Pop the seeds into a measuring cup and set aside.

Peel the orange and divide into wedges. Set aside.

Now, process lime, zucchini, kiwi, pomegranate seeds, and orange in a juicer.

Transfer to a serving glasses and add some ice cubes before serving.

Nutritional information per serving: Kcal: 183, Protein: 8.5g, Carbs: 52.6g, Fats: 1.6g

41. Guava Cucumber Juice

Ingredients:

1 cup guava, chopped

1 large cucumber, sliced

1 cup pineapple, chopped

2 large limes, peeled

1 tbsp fresh mint, chopped

2 oz water

Preparation:

Wash the guava and cut into chunks. Fill the measuring cup and reserve the rest for some other recipe in a refrigerator.

Wash the cucumber and cut into thin slices. Set aside.

Cut the top of a pineapple and peel it using a sharp knife. Cut into small chunks and fill the measuring cup. Reserve the rest of the pineapple in a refrigerator.

Peel the limes and cut lengthwise in half. Set aside.

Now, combine guava, cucumber, pineapple, limes, and mint in a juicer. Process until well juiced and transfer to serving glasses. Stir in the water and refrigerate for 15 minutes before serving.

Nutritional information per serving: Kcal: 158, Protein: 4.7g, Carbs: 47.9g, Fats: 1.1g

42. Cucumber Plum Juice

Ingredients:

1 large cucumber, sliced

5 large plums, pitted

1 cup blackberries

1 cup green cabbage, chopped

2 oz water

Preparation:

Wash the cucumber and cut into thin slices. Set aside.

Wash the plums and cut in half. Remove the pits and cut into quarters. Set aside.

Rinse the blackberries under cold running water using a colander. Slightly drain and set aside.

Wash the cabbage thoroughly under cold running water. Drain and roughly chop it. Set aside.

Now, combine cucumber, plums, blackberries, and cabbage in a juicer and process until juice. Transfer to serving glasses and stir in the water. Refrigerate for 10 minutes before serving.

Nutritional information per serving: Kcal: 221, Protein: 7.5g, Carbs: 69.1g, Fats: 2.1g

43. Grapefruit Banana Juice

Ingredients:

1 whole grapefruit, peeled

1 large banana, peeled

1 cup mango, cut into chunks

1 cup fresh mint, roughly chopped

2 large strawberries, chopped

Preparation:

Peel the grapefruit and divide into wedges. Cut each wedge in half and set aside.

Peel the banana and cut into small pieces. Set aside.

Peel the mango and cut into small chunks. Fill the measuring cup and reserve the rest in the refrigerator. Set aside.

Rinse the mint roughly and torn with hands. Set aside.

Wash the strawberries and remove the stems. Cut into bite-sized pieces and set aside.

Now, combine grapefruit, banana, mango, mint, and strawberries in a juicer and process until juiced. Transfer to a serving glass and add some ice cubes before serving.

Enjoy!

Nutritional information per serving: Kcal: 301, Protein: 5.9g, Carbs: 88.5g, Fats: 1.7g

44. Lime Apple Juice

Ingredients:

1 whole lime, peeled

1 small Granny Smith's apple, cored

1 cup celery, chopped

1 cup fresh kale, torn

1 cup fresh mint, torn

Preparation:

Peel the lime and cut into small pieces. Set aside.

Wash the apple and cut in half. Remove the core and cut into bite-sized pieces. Set aside.

Combine kale and mint in a large colander. Wash thoroughly under cold running water. Slightly drain and torn with hands. Set aside.

Wash the celery and chop into small pieces. Fill the measuring cup and set aside.

Now, combine kale, mint, celery, lime, and apple in a juicer and process until juiced. Transfer to a serving glass and add some ice before serving.

Enjoy!

Nutritional information per serving: Kcal: 121, Protein: 5.3g, Carbs: 35.8g, Fats: 1.3g

ADDITIONAL TITLES FROM THIS AUTHOR

70 Effective Meal Recipes to Prevent and Solve Being Overweight: Burn Fat Fast by Using Proper Dieting and Smart Nutrition

By Joe Correa CSN

48 Acne Solving Meal Recipes: The Fast and Natural Path to Fixing Your Acne Problems in Less Than 10 Days!

By Joe Correa CSN

41 Alzheimer's Preventing Meal Recipes: Reduce or Eliminate Your Alzheimer's Condition in 30 Days or Less!

By Joe Correa CSN

70 Effective Breast Cancer Meal Recipes: Prevent and Fight Breast Cancer with Smart Nutrition and Powerful Foods

By Joe Correa CSN

CPSIA information can be obtained
at www.ICGtesting.com
Printed in the USA
BVHW041201171120
593537BV00016B/236